KEGEL EXERCISES FOR MEN

A Comprehensive Guide On Addressing Male Pelvic Health Through Kegel Exercises With Kegels And Vaginal Training For Men's Health

CONTENTS

INTRODUCTION

Welcome to "Unlocking Vitality: The Ultimate Guide to Kegel Exercises for Men," where we embark on a transformative journey towards optimal pelvic floor health. In this book, we delve into the often overlooked yet crucial aspect of men's wellness – the pelvic floor.

A. Brief overview of pelvic floor health issues in men:

The pelvic floor, a complex network of muscles, ligaments, and tissues, plays a pivotal role in maintaining urinary and sexual function, as well as providing support to the organs within the pelvis. Despite its significance, pelvic floor health is frequently disregarded in men's health discussions. However, issues such as urinary incontinence, erectile dysfunction, and pelvic pain underscore the importance of addressing pelvic floor dysfunction in men.

B. Importance of Kegel exercises, vaginal training, and relaxation techniques:

Enter Kegel exercises – a simple yet powerful solution to bolster pelvic floor strength and function. Through targeted exercises aimed at strengthening the muscles of the pelvic floor, men can regain control over bladder function, enhance sexual performance, and alleviate pelvic discomfort. Moreover, integrating vaginal training and relaxation techniques into the regimen offers comprehensive support for pelvic floor health, fostering a harmonious balance within the body.

C. Promise of avoiding surgery through proactive pelvic floor care:

By embracing proactive pelvic floor care through Kegel exercises and associated techniques, men can potentially sidestep the need for invasive surgical interventions. Rather than resorting to surgical procedures as a reactive measure, this book advocates for a proactive approach that empowers individuals to take charge of their pelvic floor health, reclaiming vitality and vitality without the risks and recovery associated with surgery.

In "Unlocking Vitality," we embark on a journey towards renewed vigor, vitality, and confidence by unlocking the potential of Kegel exercises and holistic pelvic floor care. Join me as we discover the transformative power of proactive pelvic floor maintenance and embark on a path towards lifelong wellness and vitality.

UNDERSTANDING PELVIC FLOOR DYSFUNCTION

In the intricate architecture of the human body, there exists a silent hero often overlooked—the pelvic floor. Nestled at the base of our pelvis, this intricate web of muscles plays a pivotal role in maintaining continence, supporting pelvic organs, and facilitating sexual function. Yet, despite its significance, many remain unaware of its existence until they encounter dysfunction.

A. The Pelvic Floor: Foundation of Stability and Function:

Imagine the pelvic floor as a hammock, cradling vital organs such as the bladder, rectum, and in men, the prostate. Comprised of muscles, ligaments, and connective tissues, this dynamic structure offers stability to the pelvis while allowing flexibility for essential functions like urination, defecation, and sexual activity.

The muscles of the pelvic floor can be divided into two layers: superficial and deep. The superficial muscles, including the bulbospongiosus and ischiocavernosus, aid in erectile function and ejaculation. Meanwhile, the deeper muscles, such as the pubococcygeus and puborectalis, support the pelvic organs and contribute to urinary and fecal continence.

B. Common Pelvic Floor Disorders in Men:

Despite its resilience, the pelvic floor is susceptible to dysfunction, manifesting in various forms:

1. Incontinence: Often associated with aging or prostate surgery, urinary incontinence in men can range from mild leakage to complete loss of bladder control. Stress incontinence, characterized by urine leakage during physical exertion, and urge incontinence, marked by a sudden, intense need to urinate, are prevalent among men with pelvic floor issues.

2. Constipation: Difficulty in passing stool or incomplete bowel movements can stem from pelvic floor dysfunction. When the

muscles fail to relax properly during defecation, it hampers the expulsion of waste, leading to discomfort and strain.

3. Pelvic Pain: Chronic pelvic pain syndrome is a complex condition marked by persistent discomfort in the pelvic region. While its exact cause remains elusive, pelvic floor dysfunction is often implicated, contributing to sensations of pressure, burning, or discomfort during urination, bowel movements, or sexual activity.

C. Impact on Quality of Life and Mental Well-being:

The repercussions of pelvic floor dysfunction extend beyond physical discomfort, profoundly affecting one's quality of life and mental well-being. Coping with urinary or fecal incontinence can be emotionally distressing, leading to embarrassment, social withdrawal, and diminished self-esteem. Moreover, chronic pelvic pain can disrupt daily activities, strain relationships, and exacerbate feelings of anxiety or depression.

For many men, the silent struggle with pelvic floor dysfunction remains shrouded in stigma and misconceptions. Yet, understanding the intricacies of this vital anatomical structure and its potential ailments is the first step toward reclaiming control and seeking effective solutions.

THE SCIENCE BEHIND KEGEL EXERCISES

A. What are Kegel exercises?

Kegel exercises, named after Dr. Arnold Kegel who first introduced them in the 1940s, are a series of pelvic floor muscle contractions aimed at strengthening the muscles that support the bladder, rectum, and urethra. These exercises primarily target the pubococcygeus (PC) muscles, which play a crucial role in controlling urinary and bowel functions, as well as sexual function.

B. How do Kegel exercises strengthen the pelvic floor muscles?

The pelvic floor muscles, like any other muscle group in the body, can be strengthened through regular exercise. Kegel exercises involve contracting and relaxing the pelvic floor muscles repeatedly. This contraction and relaxation action increases blood flow to the pelvic region, promoting muscle growth and endurance over time.

When performed correctly, Kegel exercises engage the PC muscles, which are responsible for controlling the flow of urine and maintaining bowel continence. Strengthening these muscles can help prevent or alleviate issues such as urinary incontinence, fecal incontinence, and pelvic organ prolapse. Additionally, stronger pelvic floor muscles can enhance sexual function by improving erection quality and ejaculatory control.

C. Benefits of Kegel exercises for men's health:

The benefits of Kegel exercises extend beyond urinary and sexual health. For men, incorporating Kegel exercises into their fitness routine can lead to:

1. Improved urinary control: Strengthening the pelvic floor muscles can help reduce symptoms of urinary incontinence,

such as leakage or sudden urges to urinate.

2. Enhanced sexual function: By increasing blood flow to the pelvic region and improving muscle control, Kegel exercises can contribute to better erectile function, increased ejaculatory control, and more intense orgasms.

3. Prevention of pelvic organ prolapse: Pelvic organ prolapse occurs when the pelvic organs, such as the bladder, uterus, or rectum, bulge into the vaginal wall or descend into the pelvic cavity. Strengthening the pelvic floor muscles with Kegel exercises can

help support these organs and reduce the risk of prolapse.

4. Relief from pelvic pain: Kegel exercises may help alleviate symptoms of chronic pelvic pain syndrome by improving muscle strength and reducing tension in the pelvic floor.

D. Practical tips for performing Kegel exercises correctly:

To reap the full benefits of Kegel exercises, it's essential to perform them correctly. Here are some practical tips:

1. Identify the correct muscles: Before starting Kegel exercises, it's crucial to identify the pelvic floor

muscles. One way to do this is by stopping the flow of urine midstream. The muscles used to accomplish this are the ones targeted by Kegel exercises.

2. Start slowly: Begin with a few repetitions of Kegel exercises each day, gradually increasing the number of repetitions as the muscles become stronger.

3. Focus on form: When performing Kegel exercises, focus on contracting the pelvic floor muscles without tensing the muscles in the abdomen, buttocks, or thighs. Hold each contraction for a few seconds before releasing.

4. Be consistent: Like any exercise routine, consistency is key to seeing results. Aim to incorporate Kegel exercises into your daily routine, whether it's during your morning routine, while sitting at your desk, or before going to bed.

By understanding the science behind Kegel exercises and following these practical tips, men can take proactive steps towards improving their pelvic floor health and overall well-being.

VAGINAL TRAINING FOR MEN: BREAKING STEREOTYPES

In the realm of pelvic floor health, there exists a widely-held misconception: that vaginal training is exclusively for women. This myth not only perpetuates gender stereotypes but also deprives men of a valuable tool for pelvic floor rehabilitation and overall wellness. In this chapter, we will dispel these myths, delve into the benefits of vaginal training for men, and explore tailored techniques and exercises to engage in this practice effectively.

A.   Dispelling Myths and Misconceptions:

The notion that vaginal training is only for women is deeply ingrained in societal attitudes and perceptions. This misconception stems from a fundamental misunderstanding of anatomy and physiology. Contrary to popular belief, the pelvic floor muscles are not exclusive to any gender. Both men and women have pelvic floor muscles that support the bladder, bowel, and sexual function.

By perpetuating the myth that vaginal training is solely for women, we inadvertently reinforce harmful stereotypes and hinder men from seeking help for pelvic floor issues. It's time to challenge these misconceptions and recognize that vaginal training can benefit everyone, regardless of gender.

B. Explanation of How Vaginal Training Aids in Pelvic Floor Rehabilitation:

Pelvic floor rehabilitation is crucial for maintaining urinary and bowel continence, supporting sexual function, and preventing pelvic organ prolapse. Vaginal training, often associated with women's health, plays a pivotal role in pelvic floor rehabilitation for men as well.

Engaging in vaginal training allows men to strengthen and tone their pelvic floor muscles, improving bladder and bowel control, enhancing sexual performance, and reducing the risk of pelvic floor disorders. By incorporating vaginal training into their pelvic floor rehabilitation routine, men can address issues such as urinary incontinence, erectile dysfunction, and pelvic pain with greater efficacy.

C. Techniques and Exercises Tailored for Men:

Vaginal training for men involves techniques and exercises specifically designed to target the pelvic floor muscles. While the terminology may suggest otherwise, these exercises do not require access to a vagina and can be performed by men independently.

1. Kegel Exercises: Kegels involve contracting and relaxing the pelvic floor muscles to strengthen them. To perform Kegels, men can imagine stopping the flow of urine midstream or tightening the muscles used to prevent passing gas. Hold the contraction for a few seconds before releasing and repeating.

2. Reverse Kegels: Reverse Kegels focus on relaxing the pelvic floor muscles rather than contracting them. This can help alleviate tension and improve pelvic floor function. To perform reverse Kegels, men can practice consciously releasing and relaxing the pelvic floor muscles while breathing deeply.

3. Pelvic Floor Biofeedback: Biofeedback techniques utilize devices or apps to provide real-time feedback on pelvic floor muscle activity. This allows men to monitor their progress and ensure they are engaging the correct muscles during exercises.

4. Pelvic Floor Physical Therapy: For men experiencing pelvic floor dysfunction, seeking the guidance of a pelvic floor physical therapist can be immensely beneficial. These professionals can provide personalized treatment plans, including manual therapy techniques and tailored exercises to address specific concerns.

TROUBLESHOOTING AND COMMON PITFALLS

Embarking on a journey to improve pelvic health through Kegel exercises is commendable, but it's essential to navigate potential obstacles and pitfalls along the way. In this chapter, we'll explore common challenges that men may encounter during their Kegel exercise regimen and provide strategies for troubleshooting effectively.

A. Overcoming challenges and barriers to consistency:

Consistency is key to reaping the benefits of Kegel exercises. However, life's demands often pose challenges that can derail your commitment to regular practice. Whether it's a busy schedule, forgetfulness, or simply feeling unmotivated, there are strategies to overcome these barriers:

1. Establish a Routine: Incorporate Kegel exercises into your daily routine, such as performing them during your morning or evening rituals. Set reminders on your phone or calendar to ensure you don't forget.

2. Start Small: If finding time for lengthy exercise sessions is difficult, break your routine into shorter, more manageable segments. Even a few minutes of

Kegel exercises each day can make a difference.

3. Stay Motivated: Set realistic goals and track your progress to stay motivated. Celebrate small victories along the way, whether it's increased endurance or improved bladder control.

4. Enlist Support: Share your goals with a supportive friend, partner, or healthcare professional who can offer encouragement and accountability.

B. Recognizing signs of overexertion or incorrect technique:

While Kegel exercises are beneficial when performed correctly, overexertion or incorrect technique can lead to discomfort or even injury. It's crucial to listen to your body and recognize signs that you may be pushing too hard or performing the exercises incorrectly:

1. Muscle Fatigue: Feeling fatigued or sore after performing Kegel exercises is normal, but excessive fatigue may indicate overexertion. Give your muscles time to rest and recover between sessions.

2. Straining: If you find yourself straining or holding your breath while performing Kegels, you may be using incorrect technique.

Focus on engaging the pelvic floor muscles without tensing other muscles or holding your breath.

3. Discomfort: Mild discomfort or aching during Kegel exercises is common, but sharp or persistent pain is not. If you experience sharp pain, stop the exercise immediately and consult a healthcare professional.

4. Lack of Progress: If you're not seeing progress despite consistent practice, you may need to reassess your technique or consult a professional for guidance.

C. Dealing with discomfort or pain during exercises:

While discomfort during Kegel exercises is normal, it's essential to distinguish between discomfort that indicates progress and pain that signals a problem. Here are some strategies for managing discomfort during exercises:

1. Modify Your Technique: Experiment with different positions and techniques to find what works best for you. Relaxing the surrounding muscles and focusing on isolating the pelvic floor can help reduce discomfort.

2. Take Breaks: If you're experiencing discomfort or fatigue, take breaks during your exercise sessions. Gradually increase the duration and intensity

of your exercises as your muscles strengthen.

3. Use Props: Props such as pillows or cushions can provide support and make Kegel exercises more comfortable, especially if you're experiencing discomfort while sitting or lying down.

4. Consult a Professional: If you're experiencing persistent or severe pain during Kegel exercises, seek guidance from a healthcare professional. They can assess your technique, provide personalized recommendations, and address any underlying issues contributing to your discomfort.

D. Seeking professional guidance when necessary:

While Kegel exercises can be beneficial for many men, there are instances where professional guidance may be necessary to ensure safety and effectiveness:

1. Pre-existing Conditions: If you have pre-existing pelvic health conditions such as pelvic pain, urinary incontinence, or erectile dysfunction, consult a healthcare professional before starting Kegel exercises. They can tailor a program to address your specific needs and concerns.

2. Difficulty Performing Exercises: If you're having difficulty performing Kegel exercises or

aren't seeing the desired results, consider seeking guidance from a pelvic health physical therapist or urologist. They can assess your pelvic floor function, provide hands-on guidance, and recommend appropriate modifications.

3. Persistent Pain or Discomfort: If you experience persistent pain or discomfort during Kegel exercises, don't ignore it. Consult a healthcare professional to rule out any underlying issues and receive appropriate treatment.

INTEGRATING KEGEL EXERCISES INTO A HEALTHY LIFESTYLE

In our journey toward optimal pelvic floor health, it's crucial to understand that Kegel exercises are just one piece of the puzzle. To truly enhance pelvic floor function and overall well-being, we must integrate these exercises into a holistic approach to men's health. This chapter explores the importance of dietary considerations, regular physical activity, and other lifestyle factors in fostering a robust pelvic floor and overall wellness.

A. Dietary Considerations for Pelvic Floor Health:

What we consume has a profound impact on every aspect of our health, including the strength and function of our pelvic floor muscles. Incorporating certain dietary habits can support pelvic floor health and optimize the effectiveness of Kegel exercises. Here are some key considerations:

1. IIydration: Adequate hydration is essential for maintaining optimal muscle function, including the muscles of the pelvic floor. Aim to drink plenty of water throughout the day to ensure proper hydration.

2. Fiber-Rich Foods: Constipation and straining during bowel movements can strain the pelvic

floor muscles. Consuming a diet rich in fiber from fruits, vegetables, whole grains, and legumes can promote regular bowel movements and reduce the risk of pelvic floor dysfunction.

3. Balanced Diet: Opt for a balanced diet that includes a variety of nutrient-dense foods, such as lean proteins, healthy fats, fruits, and vegetables. Certain nutrients, such as magnesium and potassium, play a role in muscle function and may benefit pelvic floor health.

4. Limiting Irritants: Some individuals may find that certain foods and beverages, such as caffeine, spicy foods, and acidic

foods, can irritate the bladder and contribute to urinary symptoms. Pay attention to how your body responds to different foods and consider reducing or avoiding potential irritants.

B. Importance of Regular Physical Activity and Overall Fitness:

In addition to targeted pelvic floor exercises like Kegels, maintaining an active lifestyle is essential for promoting pelvic floor health and overall well-being. Regular physical activity offers a multitude of benefits, including:

1.   Strengthening Muscles: Engaging in activities that target the core and pelvic floor muscles, such as walking, swimming, yoga,

and Pilates, can help strengthen these muscle groups and improve their function.

2. Improving Circulation: Physical activity promotes blood flow throughout the body, including to the pelvic region. Improved circulation can support the health and vitality of pelvic tissues and muscles.

3. Weight Management: Maintaining a healthy weight through regular exercise can reduce the risk of pelvic floor disorders, such as urinary incontinence and pelvic organ prolapse, which are more prevalent in individuals who are overweight or obese.

4. Enhancing Mood and Mental Health: Exercise releases endorphins, which can help alleviate stress, anxiety, and depression. Mental well-being is closely linked to physical health, and incorporating regular exercise into your routine can have profound benefits for both body and mind.

C. Other Lifestyle Factors Affecting Pelvic Floor Function:

In addition to diet and exercise, several other lifestyle factors can impact pelvic floor function. These include:

1. Posture: Maintaining good posture throughout the day can help alleviate pressure on the

pelvic floor and prevent dysfunction. Be mindful of your posture when sitting, standing, and lifting objects.

2. Stress Management: Chronic stress can contribute to pelvic floor tension and dysfunction. Incorporate stress-reducing practices such as mindfulness, meditation, deep breathing exercises, and relaxation techniques into your daily routine.

3. Smoking Cessation: Smoking has been linked to pelvic floor disorders, including urinary incontinence. If you smoke, quitting can improve bladder function and overall pelvic floor health.

D. Creating a Holistic Approach to Men's Health and Well-being:

Optimal health is not just about the absence of disease but encompasses physical, mental, and emotional well-being. By adopting a holistic approach to men's health, we can address the interconnectedness of various factors that influence pelvic floor function and overall wellness.

1. Regular Health Screenings: Schedule regular check-ups with your healthcare provider to monitor your overall health and address any concerns or symptoms related to pelvic floor function.

2. Open Communication: Discuss any pelvic floor issues or concerns with your healthcare provider openly and honestly. They can provide guidance, support, and personalized recommendations tailored to your individual needs.

3. Self-care Practices: Incorporate self-care practices into your daily routine to nurture your physical, mental, and emotional well-being. This may include adequate sleep, relaxation techniques, hobbies, and activities that bring you joy and fulfillment.

RELAXATION TECHNIQUES FOR PELVIC FLOOR HEALTH

In the journey towards optimal pelvic floor health, one of the most crucial yet often overlooked aspects is relaxation. The intricate network of muscles and tissues comprising the pelvic floor can become tense and strained due to various factors such as stress, poor posture, or habitual muscle tightening. In this chapter, we delve into the significance of relaxation in managing pelvic floor dysfunction and explore practical techniques to achieve it.

A. Importance of relaxation in managing pelvic floor dysfunction:

Imagine your pelvic floor as a complex system of muscles, akin to a finely tuned instrument. Just as tension in a guitar string affects its ability to produce harmonious sounds, tension in the pelvic floor muscles can disrupt their function and lead to a myriad of issues such as urinary incontinence, erectile dysfunction, or pelvic pain.

Relaxation serves as the antidote to this tension, allowing the pelvic floor muscles to return to their natural state of balance and flexibility. By learning to release chronic tension and stress held within the pelvic floor, individuals can alleviate symptoms of dysfunction and promote overall well-being.

B. Mindfulness, breathing exercises, and meditation for pelvic floor relaxation:

One of the most effective ways to cultivate relaxation in the pelvic floor is through mindfulness practices such as deep breathing and meditation. These techniques not only calm the mind but also facilitate a profound connection with the body, enabling individuals to consciously release tension from the pelvic floor muscles.

Begin by finding a quiet space where you can sit or lie down comfortably. Close your eyes and bring your attention to your breath, allowing it to flow naturally in and out of your body. As you inhale, envision the breath gently expanding your pelvic floor, creating space and openness. With each exhale, release any tension or tightness you may be holding in the pelvic region, allowing the muscles to soften and relax.

Incorporating mindfulness into daily life can also help maintain pelvic floor health. Whether you're sitting at your desk, driving in traffic, or standing in line at the grocery store, take moments throughout the day to check in with your pelvic floor and consciously release any tension you may be holding.

C. Integrating relaxation practices into daily routines for optimal results:

Achieving lasting pelvic floor relaxation requires consistency and commitment. Rather than viewing relaxation as a separate task to be checked off your to-do list, integrate it seamlessly into your daily routines.

For example, you can practice deep breathing exercises while waiting for your morning coffee to brew or incorporate brief moments of mindfulness into your daily commute. Consider setting reminders on your phone or placing sticky notes in prominent locations as gentle prompts to prioritize pelvic floor relaxation throughout the day.

Additionally, exploring complementary practices such as yoga or tai chi can further enhance pelvic floor health by promoting overall body awareness and relaxation.

By making relaxation a priority and weaving it into the fabric of your daily life, you can unlock the key to optimal pelvic floor health and reclaim vitality and vitality.

OVERCOMING INCONTINENCE WITH KEGEL EXERCISES

Urinary incontinence, a condition often associated with embarrassment and discomfort, affects countless men worldwide. Whether it's a slight leakage with laughter or a more significant issue requiring pads or protective garments, the impact on one's quality of life can be profound. However, there's hope. In this chapter, we delve into the types and causes of urinary incontinence in men, explore the pivotal role of Kegel exercises and relaxation techniques in managing and preventing incontinence, and share inspiring real-life success stories of men who have triumphed over this condition through pelvic floor exercises.

A. Types and Causes of Urinary Incontinence in Men:

Urinary incontinence isn't a one-size-fits-all condition. There are various types, each with its own set of causes and characteristics. Understanding these distinctions is crucial for effective management and treatment.

1. Stress Incontinence: This type of incontinence occurs when pressure is exerted on the bladder, leading to leakage. Activities such as laughing, coughing, sneezing, or lifting heavy objects can trigger stress incontinence. Weakness in the pelvic floor muscles, often due

to factors like prostate surgery, obesity, or aging, is a common cause.

2. Urge Incontinence: Also known as overactive bladder, urge incontinence involves a sudden, intense urge to urinate followed by involuntary bladder contractions and leakage. Neurological conditions, such as Parkinson's disease or multiple sclerosis, and bladder irritants like caffeine or alcohol, can contribute to this type of incontinence.

3. Overflow Incontinence: Characterized by frequent or constant dribbling of urine, overflow incontinence occurs when the bladder doesn't empty

completely. Causes include an enlarged prostate, nerve damage from diabetes, or medications that affect bladder function.

4. Functional Incontinence: In some cases, physical or cognitive impairments prevent men from reaching the bathroom in time, leading to functional incontinence. Conditions such as arthritis, dementia, or mobility issues can contribute to this form of incontinence.

B. Role of Kegel Exercises and Relaxation in Managing and Preventing Incontinence:

While the causes and types of urinary incontinence may vary, one common thread in managing and preventing this condition is strengthening the pelvic floor muscles through Kegel exercises. These exercises, originally developed by Dr. Arnold Kegel in the 1940s, target the muscles that support the bladder, urethra, and rectum, ultimately improving bladder control and reducing leakage.

Kegel exercises involve contracting and relaxing the pelvic floor muscles, akin to the motion of stopping the flow of urine midstream. Regular practice can lead to noticeable improvements in bladder control over time. Additionally, incorporating relaxation techniques, such as deep breathing and mindfulness, can complement Kegel exercises by reducing stress and tension in the pelvic area.

C. Real-Life Success Stories of Men Who Have Overcome Incontinence Through Pelvic Floor Exercises:

The journey to overcoming urinary incontinence is often challenging but ultimately rewarding. Real-life accounts of men who have regained control of their bladder through pelvic floor exercises serve as beacons of hope for others facing similar struggles.

Take James, for example, a 58-year-old man who experienced stress incontinence following prostate surgery. Initially embarrassed and frustrated by his leakage episodes, James dedicated himself to a regimen of daily Kegel exercises and relaxation techniques. With perseverance and patience, he gradually noticed a significant reduction in leakage until eventually achieving full continence.

Similarly, David, a 45-year-old man diagnosed with overactive bladder syndrome, found relief through a combination of Kegel exercises and lifestyle modifications. By diligently practicing pelvic floor exercises and adopting strategies to manage his triggers, such as avoiding caffeinated beverages and scheduling regular bathroom breaks, David regained control over his bladder and reclaimed his active lifestyle.

These success stories underscore the transformative power of pelvic floor exercises in overcoming urinary incontinence. While the path may be challenging, with commitment and determination, men can reclaim control of their bladder and live life to the fullest.

COMBATTING CONSTIPATION WITH KEGEL EXERCISES

A. Understanding the Link between Pelvic Floor Dysfunction and Constipation:

Constipation is a common yet often overlooked ailment that can significantly impact one's quality of life. Many individuals might not realize that the pelvic floor muscles play a crucial role in bowel movements. When these muscles are weak or dysfunctional, it can lead to difficulties in passing stool, resulting in constipation.

The pelvic floor muscles act as a supportive hammock, helping to control bowel and bladder function. When they are weak or tense, they may not effectively relax and contract during defecation, leading to incomplete emptying of the bowel and constipation. Factors such as age, childbirth, chronic straining during bowel movements, and certain medical conditions can contribute to pelvic floor dysfunction, exacerbating constipation issues.

B. How Kegel Exercises and Relaxation Techniques Alleviate Constipation:

Kegel exercises, traditionally associated with improving bladder control and sexual function, can also be beneficial in combating constipation by strengthening the pelvic floor muscles. These exercises involve contracting and relaxing the muscles used to control urination and bowel movements. When performed regularly, Kegels can enhance the coordination and strength of the pelvic floor, promoting more efficient bowel movements.

In addition to Kegel exercises, relaxation techniques such as deep breathing and mindfulness meditation can help alleviate constipation by reducing tension in the pelvic floor muscles. Chronic stress and anxiety can contribute to pelvic floor dysfunction, leading to constipation. By incorporating relaxation techniques into daily routines, individuals can promote relaxation in the pelvic area, facilitating smoother bowel movements.

C. Dietary and Lifestyle Adjustments to Support Pelvic Floor Health and Bowel Regularity:

Alongside Kegel exercises and relaxation techniques, making dietary and lifestyle adjustments can further support pelvic floor health and bowel regularity. Consuming a fiber-rich diet with plenty of fruits, vegetables, whole grains, and legumes can add bulk to stool, making it easier to pass. Adequate hydration is also essential for maintaining soft, easily passed stool.

HEALING PELVIC PAIN

A. Causes and Types of Pelvic Pain in Men:

Pelvic pain in men can be a debilitating condition, often shrouded in silence and stigma. It's crucial to understand the various causes and types of pelvic pain to effectively address and manage it.

1. Chronic Prostatitis/Chronic Pelvic Pain Syndrome (CP/CPPS): This is one of the most common types of pelvic pain in men. It is characterized by persistent pain in the pelvic region, often accompanied by urinary symptoms and sexual dysfunction.

The exact cause of CP/CPPS is not fully understood, but factors such as inflammation, muscle tension, and nerve sensitization may play a role.

2. Pelvic Floor Dysfunction: Dysfunction of the pelvic floor muscles can lead to pelvic pain. These muscles play a crucial role in supporting the pelvic organs and maintaining urinary and bowel continence. When they become tight or weak, they can cause pain and dysfunction in the pelvic region.

3. Pelvic Inflammatory Disease (PID): While PID is more commonly associated with women, men can also develop pelvic pain

due to infection or inflammation of the pelvic organs, such as the prostate, bladder, or urethra.

4. Pelvic Trauma: Trauma to the pelvic area, whether from injury, surgery, or radiation therapy, can result in chronic pelvic pain.

5. Interstitial Cystitis/Bladder Pain Syndrome (IC/BPS): Although more prevalent in women, men can also experience IC/BPS, which involves bladder pain and urinary symptoms.

Understanding the specific cause of pelvic pain is essential for tailoring an effective treatment plan.

B. Role of Kegel Exercises, Vaginal Training, and Relaxation in Relieving Pelvic Pain:

Kegel exercises, often associated with strengthening the pelvic floor muscles, can be a valuable tool in relieving pelvic pain in men. While traditionally thought of as exercises for women, men can benefit greatly from incorporating Kegels into their routine.

1. Kegel Exercises for Pelvic Floor Relaxation: Contrary to popular belief, pelvic pain in men is not always due to weak pelvic floor muscles. In many cases, the muscles may be tense and overactive, contributing to pain and dysfunction. In such cases,

Kegel exercises focused on relaxation rather than contraction can be beneficial. These exercises involve consciously relaxing the pelvic floor muscles to reduce tension and alleviate pain.

2. Vaginal Training Devices: Vaginal training devices, such as biofeedback tools or pelvic floor traincrs, can help men properly engage and relax their pelvic floor muscles. These devices provide visual or auditory feedback, allowing individuals to learn how to control their pelvic floor muscles more effectively.

3. Relaxation Techniques: Stress and tension can exacerbate pelvic pain by causing the pelvic floor

muscles to tighten further. Incorporating relaxation techniques such as deep breathing, mindfulness meditation, or progressive muscle relaxation can help reduce stress and promote relaxation in the pelvic area.

C. Holistic Approaches to Managing and Treating Chronic Pelvic Pain Without Surgery:

Managing chronic pelvic pain often requires a holistic approach that addresses physical, emotional, and lifestyle factors contributing to the condition. While surgery may be necessary in some cases, many individuals find relief through non-invasive methods.

1. Physical Therapy: Pelvic floor physical therapy, conducted by specialized therapists, focuses on restoring balance and function to the pelvic floor muscles. Techniques may include manual therapy, stretching, and exercises tailored to the individual's needs.

2. Diet and Nutrition: Certain foods and beverages can irritate the bladder and exacerbate pelvic pain symptoms. Avoiding triggers such as caffeine, alcohol, spicy foods, and acidic foods may help reduce symptoms. Additionally, staying hydrated and maintaining a balanced diet rich in fruits, vegetables, and whole grains can support overall pelvic health.

3. Stress Management: Chronic pelvic pain can be emotionally taxing, leading to anxiety, depression, and decreased quality of life. Incorporating stress management techniques such as relaxation exercises, counseling, or support groups can help individuals cope with the emotional impact of pelvic pain.

4. Complementary Therapies: Acupuncture, massage therapy, and yoga are examples of complementary therapies that some individuals find beneficial for managing pelvic pain. These approaches focus on promoting relaxation, improving circulation, and reducing muscle tension in the pelvic area.

THE PROFOUND BENEFITS OF KEGEL EXERCISES FOR MEN

As we delve deeper into the realm of Kegel exercises for men, it becomes increasingly evident that these seemingly simple pelvic floor exercises offer a myriad of benefits that extend far beyond their initial conception. In this chapter, we will explore the profound advantages that Kegel exercises bring to men, enhancing various aspects of their health and well-being.

A. Improved Bladder Control and Urinary Health:

One of the primary benefits of Kegel exercises for men lies in their ability to improve bladder control and promote urinary health. The pelvic floor muscles play a crucial role in supporting the bladder and controlling the flow of urine. However, factors such as age, obesity, and prostate issues can weaken these muscles, leading to urinary incontinence and other bladder-related problems.

By regularly engaging in Kegel exercises, men can strengthen their pelvic floor muscles, thereby enhancing their ability to control urinary function. Whether it's reducing the frequency of nocturnal urination or minimizing instances of urinary leakage, Kegel exercises empower men to regain control over their bladder and enjoy improved urinary health.

B. Enhanced Sexual Function and Performance:

In addition to benefiting urinary health, Kegel exercises have been shown to significantly enhance sexual function and performance in men. The pelvic floor muscles play a crucial role in sexual arousal, ejaculation, and orgasm. Strengthening these muscles through Kegel exercises can lead to greater sexual control, heightened sensations, and improved erectile function.

Moreover, for men experiencing issues such as erectile dysfunction or premature ejaculation, Kegel exercises offer a natural and non-invasive solution. By increasing blood flow to the pelvic region and enhancing muscle tone, these exercises can help men achieve and sustain erections more effectively, as well as prolong sexual stamina, ultimately leading to a more fulfilling and satisfying sexual experience.

C. Prevention and Management of Pelvic Floor Disorders:

Pelvic floor disorders, including pelvic organ prolapse and fecal incontinence, can significantly impact a man's quality of life and overall well-being. Fortunately, Kegel exercises serve as a proactive measure for both the prevention and management of these conditions.

By strengthening the pelvic floor muscles, Kegel exercises help to provide better support for the pelvic organs, reducing the risk of prolapse and improving bowel control. Additionally, for men already suffering from pelvic floor disorders, such as rectal prolapse or fecal incontinence, Kegel exercises can aid in symptom management and enhance pelvic floor function, offering relief and restoring a sense of control over one's body.

D. Overall Well-being and Quality of Life:

Beyond their specific physiological benefits, Kegel exercises contribute to men's overall well-being and quality of life in profound ways. A strong and healthy pelvic floor is essential for maintaining proper posture, stability, and core strength, which are vital components of physical fitness and mobility.

Furthermore, by promoting awareness and mindfulness of the pelvic region, Kegel exercises encourage a deeper connection between mind and body, fostering a sense of empowerment and self-confidence. As men incorporate these exercises into their daily routine, they often report feeling more in tune with their bodies and better equipped to address various health challenges.

CONCLUSION

"Kegel Exercises for Men" has delved into a realm of male health that often goes overlooked. Throughout this journey, we've uncovered key insights and techniques aimed at empowering men to take control of their pelvic floor health.

Firstly, we've emphasized the importance of understanding the pelvic floor muscles and their role in various bodily functions, from urinary control to sexual performance. Through detailed explanations and guided exercises, readers have learned how to identify, locate, and effectively engage these muscles.

Secondly, the book has served as a beacon of encouragement for men to prioritize their pelvic floor health. By dispelling myths and stigma surrounding male pelvic health issues, we've created a space for open dialogue and proactive care. Through consistent practice of Kegel exercises and other recommended strategies, men can take tangible steps towards improving their overall well-being.

Lastly, as we look to the future, there is hope for a world free from the limitations of pelvic floor dysfunction. By advocating for early intervention and holistic approaches to pelvic health, we can envision a society where men are empowered to seek non-invasive solutions and live their lives to the fullest.

In closing, let us remember that pelvic floor health is not a taboo topic, but rather an essential aspect of overall wellness. By embracing the insights and techniques shared in this book, men can embark on a journey towards a future where pelvic floor dysfunction is a thing of the past. Let us prioritize proactive care, embrace the power of Kegel exercises, and envision a world where pelvic health knows no bounds.

THE END

www.ingramcontent.com/pod-product-compliance
Lightning Source LLC
Chambersburg PA
CBHW071214260726

48653CB00041B/755